SLEEP SMARTER TONIGHT: MASTER THE ART OF FALLING, STAYING RESTED, AND WAKING ENERGIZED

Proven Strategies to Enhance Sleep, Supercharge Health and Maximize Daily Performance

Caleb Franklin

Caleb Franklin

TABLE OF CONTENTS

Caleb Franklin

Chapter 4: Nutrition and Sleep

Chapter 5: Exercise and Sleep

Chapter 6: Managing Stress for Better Sleep

Chapter 7: Creating the Perfect Sleep Environment

Caleb Franklin

Chapter 8: The Psychological Aspects of Sleep

➤ Understanding Stress and Anxiety
- How Anxiety Impacts Sleep Quality
- Identifying Negative Thought Patterns

➤ Techniques for Cultivating a Positive Sleep Mindset
- Cognitive Behavioral Strategies for Better Sleep
- Visualization and Affirmation Practices

Chapter 9: Embracing Rest and Recovery

☐ The Importance of Rest Beyond Sleep
- Understanding Different Types of Rest
- Balancing Activity and Recovery

☐ Incorporating Rest into Your Daily Routine
- Practical Tips for Scheduling Rest Breaks
- Mindfulness and Relaxation Techniques Throughout the Day

Conclusion………………………………………………

☐ Your Journey to Restorative Sleep
- Recap of Key Insights and Strategies
- Encouragement for the Reader's Sleep Journey

➤ Embracing the Transformative Power of Sleep
- Long-Term Benefits of Prioritizing Sleep
- Final Thoughts and Next Steps

Caleb Franklin

Introduction:

It's another restless night. You've tried everything—counting sheep, adjusting your position for the hundredth time, scrolling through your phone in hopes of tricking yourself into sleep. But here you are, wide awake, exhausted, and frustrated. The minutes on the clock blur into hours, and before you know it, your alarm jolts you into yet another day of dragging yourself through life on empty.

Sound familiar?

Maybe you're telling yourself, "It's just the way life is now," accepting the constant fatigue as normal. After all, with everything on your plate, who has time to sleep, right? But deep down, there's a nagging thought: *There must be something wrong. * Why is it so hard for you to fall asleep when you're so tired? Why do you keep waking up in the middle of the night, staring at the ceiling, counting down the hours until morning? And why, even when you do manage to sleep, do you wake up feeling as if you never rested at all?

The truth is, you *know* something's off. And here's the thing—you're absolutely right.

What if I told you that you don't have to accept sleepless nights and groggy mornings as your new reality? That the solution to your exhaustion isn't a distant dream, but something you can grasp right now—something real, simple, and backed by science?

You're not broken. You're not doomed to live with chronic fatigue. You're just missing the right tools to fix your sleep.

Caleb Franklin

This book was written for you, the person who's tried everything and still finds themselves awake at night, the person who wakes up tired no matter how many hours they log in bed. You've been searching for answers, and you're about to find them.

You're about to discover why your current sleep habits aren't working and how you can start falling asleep faster, staying asleep longer, and waking up with the energy to power through your day like never before. And let's be clear—this isn't vague advice like "relax" or "get eight hours." This is a science-based, proven strategy that gets to the root of your sleep struggles.

Have you ever wondered what it would be like to wake up *refreshed*, without the dread of dragging yourself out of bed? Have you imagined a life where you feel energized throughout the day, focused, and ready to take on anything? It's possible. Not just for others, but for you. Right here. Right now.

Here's what you're about to uncover:

- Why your mind keeps racing when your head hits the pillow, and how to silence the noise.
- The real reason you toss and turn, and the steps to finally stay asleep all night.
- Why your sleep cycles are broken—and the simple shifts you can make to reset them.
- How to create an environment that actually promotes deep, restorative sleep.
- The sleep-inducing habits that will have you waking up refreshed, not groggy.

Caleb Franklin

No more quick fixes that fizzle out. No more sleepless nights filled with frustration. Say goodbye to waking up feeling like you haven't slept a bit. This book will walk you through the proven methods that countless others have used to conquer their sleep issues and wake up feeling alive again.

Imagine it—your mornings, not filled with groggy yawns and sluggish movements, but with clarity, energy, and enthusiasm. Picture yourself at the end of the day, winding down without stress or anxiety, knowing that restful, peaceful sleep is just around the corner. This isn't wishful thinking; it's a reality you can achieve.

The missing piece isn't some complicated formula. It's understanding the science of sleep and applying easy, actionable steps to unlock your body's natural ability to rest. Everything you need to transform your sleep—and your life—is within reach.

So, let's begin. No more sleepless nights, no more settling for exhaustion. Let's fix your sleep for good.

Every solution in this book is grounded in real science—proven methods that work for real people, just like you. I've done the research, so you don't have to. I've sifted through the countless myths, half-truths, and quick-fix solutions to bring you what actually works. No gimmicks, no fluff—just real, tangible steps that will get you from restless to rested.

So, are you ready to stop tossing and turning? Are you ready to wake up refreshed, energized, and ready to take on the day?

Caleb Franklin

This isn't about dreaming of a better night's sleep anymore. It's about making it happen. And it starts right here, right now.

Caleb Franklin

Caleb Franklin

Chapter 1: Understanding Sleep

Sleep is often treated like an afterthought—a necessary but inconvenient part of life that we try to reduce as much as possible. We're conditioned to believe that less sleep equals more productivity, more success, and more time to do the things we want. But what if everything you thought you knew about sleep was wrong?

You're here because you know that something isn't working. Maybe you're tired of feeling groggy throughout the day, pushing through fatigue just to make it to the end. Or maybe you've noticed that no matter how many hours you spend in bed, you wake up feeling like you've barely rested. And yet, you keep moving forward, because, well, that's life, right?

Wrong.

The truth is, sleep is the foundation upon which every aspect of your wellbeing is built. Your body, mind, and even your spirit rely on it. Without proper rest, you can't function at your best—physically, mentally, or emotionally. In fact, lack of sleep could be the very reason you're struggling in ways you haven't even realized yet.

Let's start by unraveling the mystery of sleep itself.

What Is Sleep, Really?

Most people think of sleep as simply a time when the body shuts down, like turning off a computer. But sleep isn't about powering off—it's about recharging.

Caleb Franklin

Sleep is an incredibly dynamic process, where your body and brain engage in essential maintenance tasks that can't happen while you're awake.

During sleep, your brain processes and organizes all the information you took in throughout the day, strengthening your memory and clearing out unnecessary clutter. Meanwhile, your body repairs damaged tissues, replenishes energy reserves, and regulates hormones that control everything from hunger to mood. In fact, sleep is so critical that going without it for too long can be more dangerous than going without food.

When you start to think of sleep as the engine behind everything your body and mind need to thrive, it becomes clear that it's not just about closing your eyes and resting. It's about setting the stage for success in every other area of your life.

Sleep Stages: How Deep Sleep and REM Restore Your Body and Mind

To truly understand the importance of sleep, we need to dive into its stages—because not all sleep is created equal. Every night, your body cycles through four main stages of sleep, each with its own unique purpose.

1.   **Light Sleep (Stage 1 & Stage 2):** This is where you begin to drift off. Your muscles relax, your heart rate slows, and your brainwaves begin to transition from active to calm. But while it feels like you're just dozing off, this phase is crucial for transitioning into deeper sleep. If you wake up during this stage, you'll feel like you barely slept at all.

2.   **Deep Sleep (Stage 3):** This is the holy grail of physical restoration. During deep sleep, your body focuses on repairing tissues, strengthening your immune

system, and rebuilding energy stores. Without enough deep sleep, you'll not only feel tired—you'll also be more vulnerable to illness, weight gain, and even chronic diseases like diabetes and heart disease.

**3.	REM Sleep (Stage 4):** This is where your brain gets its workout. REM (Rapid Eye Movement) sleep is when your brain is most active, processing emotions, solidifying memories, and clearing out unnecessary information. It's also when you dream. While it might seem like REM sleep is for your mind alone, it's just as critical for your emotional well-being. People deprived of REM sleep tend to be more irritable, anxious, and prone to mood swings.

Throughout the night, you cycle through these stages' multiple times, with each cycle becoming longer as the night progresses. This is why getting enough total sleep is so important—if you cut your sleep short, you rob yourself of crucial deep and REM sleep, leaving you feeling unrefreshed and unbalanced.

Why Sleep Is Non-Negotiable for Your Health, Productivity, and Mood

It's easy to see sleep as something you can sacrifice when life gets busy. But sacrificing sleep is like trying to drive your car without fuel—eventually, you'll break down. Here's why sleep isn't just important—it's absolutely nonnegotiable.

**1.	Health and Immunity:** When you're sleep-deprived, your immune system takes a serious hit. Sleep is when your body produces vital proteins called cytokines, which fight off infection, inflammation, and stress. Without enough sleep, your body's ability to defend itself is weakened, leaving you more susceptible to illnesses—from the common cold to serious diseases like cancer.

Caleb Franklin

2.   **Cognitive Function and Memory:** Think about the last time you pulled an all-nighter. How well were you able to concentrate the next day? Probably not well at all. That's because sleep plays a critical role in cognitive function. It's during sleep that your brain consolidates information, making it easier for you to remember and learn. Without it, you'll struggle with focus, problem-solving, and decision-making.

3.   **Emotional Balance:** Have you ever noticed how irritable and impatient you become after a bad night's sleep? Sleep and emotional regulation are intimately connected. Without enough rest, your brain has a harder time processing emotions, leading to mood swings, anxiety, and even depression. Sleep deprivation has been linked to increased risk of mental health issues, including chronic stress and burnout.

4.   **Productivity and Performance:** If you're the type who believes "I'll sleep when I'm dead," it's time to rethink that mantra. Lack of sleep directly impacts your productivity and performance in everything you do. Whether it's at work, in your relationships, or during your workouts, sleep is the fuel that powers you through each day. When you're well-rested, you'll work smarter, faster, and with more creativity and clarity.

Common Sleep Myths Debunked

There's a lot of misinformation out there about sleep, which is why so many people continue to struggle with it. Let's bust some of the most common sleep myths:

- **Myth:** You can "catch up" on sleep over the weekend.

Caleb Franklin

Reality: Sleep doesn't work like a bank account. While you may feel more rested after sleeping in on the weekend, the damage caused by chronic sleep deprivation during the week can't be fully reversed in a couple of days.

- **Myth:** Older adults need less sleep.

Reality: While sleep patterns change with age, older adults still need 7-9 hours of sleep per night. If they're getting less, it's likely due to other factors, such as health conditions or medications.

Myth: If you can't sleep, it's best to stay in bed and try harder.

Reality: If you're lying awake in bed for more than 20 minutes, it's better to get up and do something relaxing than to stay in bed stressing. This prevents your brain from linking your bed with being awake, promoting better sleep habits.

Caleb Franklin

Chapter 2: What's Sabotaging Your Sleep?

If you've ever tossed and turned through the night, you know how frustrating it can be. One minute you're drifting off, and the next, your mind is racing, thoughts swirling in a chaotic dance. You may have wondered why you're not sleeping as well as you should. What's keeping you awake? What's sabotaging your ability to get the restorative sleep you need?

In this chapter, we'll dive deep into the most common culprits that disrupt your sleep. Understanding these factors is the first step toward reclaiming your nights and transforming your days.

The Most Common Sleep Disruptors (And Why You Don't Even Notice Them)

Often, the reasons we can't sleep are subtle and insidious. You might not even realize they're impacting your ability to get a good night's rest. Let's explore some of the most common disruptors:

1.   **Stress and Anxiety:** Life can be overwhelming, and stress is a significant factor that affects our sleep quality. When you're stressed, your body produces cortisol, the stress hormone, which can keep you awake and alert when you should be winding down. If you often find your mind racing with worries about work, relationships, or the future, it's no wonder you struggle to fall asleep.

2.   **Poor Sleep Hygiene:** Your daily habits play a crucial role in your sleep quality. Irregular sleep schedules, consuming caffeine late in the day, and using your phone or computer right before bed can all lead to sleep disruptions.

Caleb Franklin

Creating a calming bedtime routine and sticking to a consistent sleep schedule are essential for improving your sleep.

3.	**Environmental Factors:** Your bedroom environment can make or break your sleep. Noise, light, and temperature can all interfere with your ability to fall asleep and stay asleep. For example, a noisy street or bright streetlights can keep you from entering those deeper sleep stages.

4.	**Diet and Lifestyle Choices:** What you eat and drink has a profound impact on your sleep. Heavy meals close to bedtime, alcohol consumption, and excessive caffeine can disrupt your sleep cycle. While alcohol might help you fall asleep faster, it often leads to fragmented sleep and lower overall quality.

5.	**Health Conditions:** Various medical issues can affect your sleep, such as sleep apnea, restless leg syndrome, and chronic pain. If you suspect that an underlying health condition is affecting your sleep, it's crucial to seek professional help.

Stress, Anxiety, and Your Racing Mind: The Silent Sleep Killers

When was the last time you laid your head down, ready to sleep, only to have your mind flood with thoughts? Stress and anxiety are among the most common reasons people experience sleep issues.

As you lie in bed, replaying the events of the day or worrying about what tomorrow may bring, your body enters a state of heightened alertness, making it nearly impossible to drift off. The more you try to force yourself to sleep, the more elusive it becomes.

Caleb Franklin

What Can You Do?

Implementing relaxation techniques before bed can help quiet your mind. Consider incorporating practices such as:

- **Mindfulness Meditation:** Spend a few minutes focusing on your breath, letting go of intrusive thoughts. Apps like Headspace or Calm offer guided meditations specifically for sleep.

- **Journaling:** Write down your thoughts, worries, or to-do lists before bed. This can help clear your mind and reduce anxiety about forgetting something important.

- **Gentle Yoga or Stretching:** Engaging in light physical activity can help release tension from your body and prepare you for sleep.

The Role of Technology and Blue Light in Destroying Your Sleep

In our digital age, it's easy to get lost in screens—whether it's scrolling through social media, binge-watching your favorite series, or catching up on emails. However, using screens before bed can severely impact your sleep quality.

The blue light emitted from devices like smartphones, tablets, and laptops interferes with your body's natural production of melatonin, the hormone that regulates sleep. When your melatonin levels are disrupted, your brain has a harder time signaling that it's time to sleep.

What Can You Do?

To combat the effects of blue light, try the following strategies:

- **Set a Digital Curfew:** Aim to turn off all screens at least 30-60 minutes before bed. Use this time to unwind with a book, practice relaxation techniques, or enjoy a warm bath.

- **Use Blue Light Filters:** If you must use screens in the evening, consider installing apps that reduce blue light exposure or using glasses designed to block blue light.

Environmental Factors That Are Robbing You of Rest

The quality of your sleep is heavily influenced by your sleep environment. Here are some key factors to consider:

1.   **Noise:** Whether it's traffic, a loud neighbor, or the hum of household appliances, noise can disrupt your sleep. Consider using white noise machines, earplugs, or soundproofing your bedroom to create a more peaceful environment.

Caleb Franklin

2.	**Light:** Exposure to light—whether from outside or from electronic devices— can interfere with your body's circadian rhythm. Use blackout curtains to block external light, and avoid bright lights in your bedroom.

3.	**Temperature:** The ideal sleep temperature is typically between 60-67°F (1519°C). An uncomfortable room temperature, whether too hot or too cold, can make it challenging to fall asleep. Consider investing in a fan or adjusting your thermostat to create a comfortable environment.

Final Thoughts on Sabotaging Your Sleep

Recognizing the factors that disrupt your sleep is the first step toward making positive changes. By identifying the culprits in your life—whether they're related to stress, technology, or your environment—you can start to reclaim your nights.

In the next chapter, we'll explore how to create an environment that promotes better sleep. You'll learn practical tips for turning your bedroom into a sleep sanctuary, allowing you to harness the restorative power of sleep and wake up refreshed, energized, and ready to tackle the day ahead.

Caleb Franklin

Chapter 3: Fixing Your Sleep Environment

Imagine stepping into a sanctuary designed just for you—a space where relaxation envelops you, and the outside world fades away. Your bedroom should be that sanctuary, a haven for rest where every element works in harmony to promote restorative sleep. If you're struggling with sleep, it might be time to evaluate your environment and make some transformative changes.

How to Create the Ultimate Sleep Sanctuary

Creating the perfect sleep environment involves more than just a comfortable bed; it's about crafting a space that calms your mind and body. Here are essential components to consider:

1.   **Comfortable Bedding:** Your mattress and pillows are the foundation of a good night's sleep. Choose a mattress that provides the right support for your body type and sleeping position. When it comes to pillows, ensure they align your head and neck comfortably. Experiment with different materials— memory foam, latex, or down—to find what suits you best.

2.   **Bedding Material:** Soft, breathable sheets can enhance your comfort. Natural materials like cotton or bamboo are great choices, as they allow for better airflow and moisture-wicking, keeping you cool throughout the night.

3.   **Organize Your Space:** A tidy environment promotes a calm and focused mindset. Take the time to tidy up your bedroom, removing distractions and creating a peaceful atmosphere. Consider storage solutions that keep your space organized while also being aesthetically pleasing.

Caleb Franklin

The Best Bedding, Mattress, and Pillow Choices for Quality Sleep

Choosing the right bedding can significantly impact your sleep quality. Here are some tips:

- **Mattress:** Look for a mattress that suits your sleep style—firm for back sleepers, medium for side sleepers, and soft for stomach sleepers. Consider trying out mattresses in stores or ordering a trial version online.

- **Pillows:** Different materials offer varying levels of support. Memory foam contours to your head and neck, while down pillows offer softness. Find one that keeps your spine aligned and prevents stiffness.

- **Duvets and Comforters:** Opt for lightweight, breathable options that can keep you warm without overheating. Consider seasonal changes and adjust your bedding accordingly.

Optimizing Light, Temperature, and Sound for Deep Sleep

Your bedroom should promote optimal conditions for sleep. Here's how to control light, temperature, and sound:

1. **Light Control:** Exposure to light signals your brain to be alert. Use blackout curtains to block out external light and consider a sleep mask for additional

darkness. Dim the lights in your home as bedtime approaches to cue your body that it's time to wind down.

2.   **Temperature Regulation:** The ideal sleep temperature is typically between 60-67°F (15-19°C). If you find yourself too hot or cold, adjust your thermostat, use fans, or invest in cooling or heating mattress pads to maintain a comfortable temperature.

3.   **Sound Management:** Noise can be a significant barrier to quality sleep. If you live in a noisy area, consider white noise machines, fans, or earplugs to drown out disruptive sounds. Additionally, calming sounds—like nature or soft music—can help you relax before bed.

Decluttering Your Space and Your Mind Before Bed

The state of your bedroom can greatly influence your mental state. An untidy space can often result in a cluttered mind. Here's how to create a calming atmosphere:

- **Create a Nightly Ritual:** Spend a few minutes each evening tidying up your bedroom. This simple act can signal to your mind that it's time to relax and prepare for sleep.

- **Limit Stimulating Activities:** In the hour leading up to bed, avoid engaging in high-energy activities or conversations that might elevate your stress levels. Instead, focus on calming routines that help transition your mind from the busyness of the day to a more restful state.

Caleb Franklin

- **Add Relaxing Elements:** Incorporate calming elements like soft lighting, soothing scents (such as lavender or chamomile), and plants that promote relaxation. Each of these can contribute to a more tranquil sleep environment.

Final Thoughts on Creating Your Sleep Sanctuary

Your bedroom should be a place that encourages rest and rejuvenation, free from distractions and stressors. By investing time and effort into creating the ultimate sleep sanctuary, you're taking a significant step toward better sleep quality and overall well-being.

In the next chapter, we'll delve into how to reset your body's internal clock, helping you fall asleep faster and wake up refreshed. You'll learn how to synchronize your sleep patterns with your natural rhythms, setting the foundation for a healthier relationship with sleep.

Caleb Franklin

Chapter 4: Resetting Your Body's Internal Clock

Have you ever noticed how some nights you drift off effortlessly while other nights feel like an uphill battle? The secret to a restful night often lies in the synchronization of your body's internal clock, known as the circadian rhythm. When this rhythm is in sync, falling asleep and waking up becomes a natural, seamless process. But when it's out of whack, sleep can feel elusive.

In this chapter, we'll explore what circadian rhythms are, how they work, and actionable strategies to reset your internal clock for better sleep.

Understanding Circadian Rhythms: The Science of Sleep Timing

Your circadian rhythm is a 24-hour internal clock that regulates your sleep wake cycle, influencing when you feel alert and when you feel sleepy. This rhythm is governed by an array of biological processes, including hormone release, body temperature, and other physiological changes.

- **Light Sensitivity:** One of the most significant influencers of your circadian rhythm is light. Natural light signals to your body that it's time to be awake, while darkness cues the production of melatonin, the hormone responsible for sleep.

- **The Role of Melatonin:** As night falls, your body starts producing melatonin, helping you feel drowsy and ready for sleep. Conversely, exposure to light—especially blue light from screens—can suppress melatonin production, delaying your ability to fall asleep.

Signs Your Internal Clock Needs Resetting

You may be wondering whether your circadian rhythm is off balance. Here are some signs to watch for:

1.   **Difficulty Falling Asleep or Waking Up:** If you find yourself staring at the ceiling for hours or waking up multiple times throughout the night, your internal clock may be misaligned.

2.   **Daytime Fatigue:** Feeling excessively tired during the day, despite spending enough hours in bed, can indicate that your sleep quality is suffering.

3.   **Mood Swings and Irritability:** Insufficient sleep can affect your mood, leading to increased irritability and anxiety.

4.   **Reliance on Caffeine or Naps:** If you're using caffeine to get through the day or relying on naps to compensate for poor sleep, it's time to reevaluate your sleep patterns.

Strategies to Reset Your Circadian Rhythm

Now that you understand what's at stake, let's explore actionable strategies to reset your internal clock and enhance your sleep quality:

Caleb Franklin

1.   Establish a Consistent Sleep Schedule: Aim to go to bed and wake up at the same time every day, even on weekends. This consistency reinforces your body's natural rhythms, making it easier to fall asleep and wake up feeling refreshed.

2.   Limit Light Exposure at Night: Create a wind-down routine that reduces exposure to bright and blue light in the hours leading up to bed. Dim the lights in your home and consider using blue light-blocking glasses if you must use screens.

3.   Get Morning Sunlight: Exposure to natural light in the morning helps reinforce your circadian rhythm. Spend time outside or near a window shortly after waking up. This signals to your body that it's time to be alert and active.

4.   Practice a Relaxing Pre-Sleep Routine: Engage in calming activities before bed to signal to your body that it's time to wind down. This might include reading, taking a warm bath, practicing gentle yoga, or engaging in mindfulness meditation.

5.   Avoid Stimulants Before Bed: Caffeine, nicotine, and even heavy meals can disrupt your ability to fall asleep. Aim to avoid these stimulants in the hours leading up to your bedtime.

6.   Limit Naps: While naps can be beneficial, they can also interfere with your nighttime sleep if taken too late in the day. If you need to nap, aim for a short 20-30-minute power nap earlier in the day.

Caleb Franklin

When to Seek Help: Recognizing Sleep Disorders

Sometimes, despite your best efforts, resetting your circadian rhythm may not be enough. If you consistently struggle with sleep issues—like insomnia, sleep apnea, or restless leg syndrome—it may be time to consult a healthcare professional. They can help identify any underlying conditions and recommend appropriate treatments.

Final Thoughts on Synchronizing Your Sleep Patterns

Resetting your body's internal clock is a powerful way to improve your sleep quality. By establishing healthy habits and being mindful of your light exposure, you can create an environment that encourages restorative rest.

In the next chapter, we'll delve into powerful techniques for enhancing your sleep quality, including relaxation strategies, breathing exercises, and the benefits of mindfulness. Together, we'll build a toolkit that empowers you to conquer sleepless nights and embrace rejuvenating rest.

Caleb Franklin

Chapter 5: Techniques for Enhancing Sleep Quality

Imagine slipping into a state of deep, restorative sleep, where your mind and body can finally recharge. The secret to achieving this level of rest lies in adopting a variety of techniques that enhance your sleep quality. In this chapter, we'll explore a range of powerful methods—from relaxation techniques to breathing exercises—that can transform your nightly routine into a sanctuary of tranquility.

The Art of Relaxation: Finding Your Calm Before Sleep

Creating a peaceful transition from the busyness of your day to the stillness of night is essential for quality sleep. Here are some effective relaxation techniques to incorporate into your nightly ritual:

1.   Guided Imagery: Visualize serene scenes that evoke feelings of peace and comfort. Picture yourself on a quiet beach, listening to the gentle waves, or walking through a tranquil forest. This mental escape can help quiet your racing mind.

2.   Progressive Muscle Relaxation: This method involves tightening and releasing each muscle group, starting from your toes and gradually moving upwards throughout your body.   This not only releases physical tension but also signals to your brain that it's time to relax.

3.   Gentle Yoga and Stretching: Engaging in gentle stretches or restorative yoga poses can alleviate physical tension and promote relaxation. Focus on your breath as you move, allowing each exhale to release any lingering stress.

Caleb Franklin

Harnessing the Power of Breath

Breathing exercises are a powerful tool for calming your mind and body, especially before bed. Here are a few techniques to explore:

1.   The 4-7-8 breathing method: developed by Dr. Andrew Weil, involves breathing in for four counts, holding for seven, and exhaling for eight, helping to promote relaxation. Repeat this cycle four times. This method helps reduce anxiety and promote relaxation.

2.   Diaphragmatic Breathing: Lie on your back with your hands on your belly. Inhale deeply through your nose, allowing your belly to rise, then exhale slowly through your mouth. Focus on the sensation of your breath, letting it anchor you to the present moment.

3.   Box Breathing: Inhale deeply for four counts, hold for four counts, exhale for four counts, and hold again for four counts. This rhythmic breathing pattern calms the nervous system and can ease tension before sleep.

Embracing Mindfulness and Meditation

Mindfulness and meditation practices can profoundly impact your sleep quality. By focusing your attention and eliminating distractions, you can cultivate a peaceful state of mind conducive to restful sleep:

1.   **Mindfulness Meditation:** Spend a few minutes each evening practicing mindfulness meditation. Sit comfortably, focus on your breath, and gently guide

Caleb Franklin

your thoughts back whenever your mind wanders. This practice trains your mind
to remain present, alleviating stress and anxiety.

2.   **Body Scan Meditation:** Lie down comfortably and bring awareness to
different parts of your body, starting from your toes and moving upward.
Notice any sensations or tension, consciously relaxing each area as you go. This
practice enhances body awareness and promotes relaxation.

3.   **Sleep Apps and Resources:** Consider using sleep meditation apps like Calm
or Insight Timer, which offer guided meditations specifically designed for sleep.
These resources can provide structure and support as you cultivate a calming pre-
sleep routine.

Creating a Sleep-Friendly Mindset

Your mindset plays a crucial role in how easily you transition into sleep. Here's
how to cultivate a sleep-friendly attitude:

1.   **Letting Go of Worries:** As bedtime approaches, write down any thoughts or
tasks on your mind. This simple act of journaling can help clear your mental slate
and reduce anxiety about forgetting something important.

2.   **Avoiding Sleep Pressure:** If you find yourself unable to sleep after 20
minutes, get out of bed and engage in a calming activity—like reading or listening
to soft music—until you feel sleepy. This prevents the frustration that can build
when you lie awake.

Caleb Franklin

3. **Cultivating Gratitude:** Incorporate a gratitude practice into your evening routine. Reflect on three things you're thankful for each day. This shift in perspective can create a sense of calm and contentment, making it easier to fall asleep.

Final Thoughts on Enhancing Sleep Quality

By integrating these relaxation techniques, breathing exercises, and mindfulness practices into your nightly routine, you can transform your sleep experience. Each method is designed to help you unwind, alleviate stress, and cultivate a sense of tranquility, allowing you to embrace the restorative power of sleep.

In the next chapter, we'll explore the fascinating relationship between nutrition and sleep, uncovering how what you eat can either enhance or hinder your sleep quality. You'll learn about foods that promote restful sleep, as well as those that might be keeping you awake at night.

Caleb Franklin

Chapter 6: The Connection Between Nutrition and Sleep

As you lay your head down each night, you may not realize the profound impact that your dietary choices have on your sleep quality. What you consume throughout the day plays a critical role in how well you rest at night. In this chapter, we'll explore the intricate relationship between nutrition and sleep, uncovering foods that promote restorative sleep and those that may keep you tossing and turning.

Understanding Sleep Nutrition: The Science Behind Food and Rest

Nutrition isn't just about calories; it's about the nutrients that fuel your body and mind. Certain foods can influence the production of sleep-related hormones, enhance your ability to fall asleep, and improve sleep quality. Understanding these connections is essential for anyone seeking to optimize their rest.

1.   **The Role of Hormones:** Serotonin, a precursor to melatonin, plays a significant role in regulating your sleep-wake cycle. Foods rich in tryptophan— an amino acid found in turkey, dairy, and nuts—can boost serotonin levels, leading to increased melatonin production.

2.   **Blood Sugar Levels:** Stable blood sugar levels throughout the day can help prevent nighttime awakenings. Foods that trigger spikes and drops in blood sugar may result in disrupted sleep. Focus on balanced meals that include complex carbohydrates, protein, and healthy fats to maintain steady energy levels.

Caleb Franklin

Foods That Promote Restful Sleep

Incorporating specific foods into your diet can help enhance your sleep quality. Here are some power players to consider:

1.   **Complex Carbohydrates:** Foods like whole grains, oats, and brown rice can help increase serotonin levels. These foods promote feelings of fullness and can enhance sleep quality when consumed in moderation.

2.   **Lean Proteins:** Incorporate lean sources of protein—such as chicken, fish, eggs, and legumes—into your meals. These proteins contain tryptophan, which supports melatonin production.

3.   **Fruits and Vegetables:** Rich in vitamins, minerals, and antioxidants, fruits and vegetables support overall health. Specific choices, such as cherries, bananas, and leafy greens, are particularly beneficial for sleep. Cherries are natural sources of melatonin, while bananas provide magnesium and potassium, which help relax muscles.

4.   **Healthy Fats:** Foods like avocados, nuts, and seeds contain omega-3 fatty acids, which can reduce inflammation and promote brain health. Healthy fats support the body's ability to absorb nutrients, enhancing overall wellness.

5.   **Herbal Teas:** Chamomile, valerian root, and lavender teas have calming properties that can aid relaxation and promote better sleep. Sipping a warm cup of herbal tea before bed can signal to your body that it's time to wind down.

Caleb Franklin

Foods to Avoid for Better Sleep

Just as some foods can enhance sleep, others may hinder your ability to rest peacefully. Here's what to avoid:

1.   **Caffeine:** Found in coffee, tea, chocolate, and many soft drinks, caffeine is a stimulant that can disrupt your sleep if consumed too close to bedtime. Aim to limit caffeine intake in the afternoon and evening.

2.   **Alcohol:** While alcohol may help you fall asleep initially, it can lead to fragmented sleep and frequent awakenings. Try to limit alcohol consumption, especially in the hours leading up to bedtime.

3.   **Heavy Meals:** Eating large, heavy meals before bed can cause discomfort and indigestion, making it difficult to fall asleep. It's best to eat your final meal two to three hours before bedtime for optimal sleep quality.

4.   **Spicy Foods:** Spicy foods can increase metabolism and body temperature, leading to discomfort during sleep. Opt for lighter, more easily digestible meals in the evening.

Creating a Sleep-Conducive Eating Schedule

When it comes to maintaining your health, the timing of your meals can be just as crucial as the foods you choose. Consider the following strategies to optimize your eating schedule for better sleep:

1.   **Regular Meal Times:** Establish a consistent eating schedule to help regulate your body's internal clock. Aim for regular meal times to keep your metabolism steady and support healthy digestion.

Caleb Franklin

2.   **Balanced Evening Meals:** Focus on balanced meals that include a mix of carbohydrates, proteins, and healthy fats. This combination can support serotonin production and keep blood sugar levels stable.

3.   **Light Snacks Before Bed:** If you find yourself hungry before sleep, opt for a light snack that combines complex carbohydrates and protein. Examples include whole-grain toast with almond butter or a small bowl of yogurt with fruit.

Hydration: The Overlooked Factor

While food plays a crucial role in sleep, hydration is equally important. Dehydration can lead to discomfort and disrupt your sleep quality. Here are some tips:

1.   **Stay Hydrated Throughout the Day:** Aim to drink plenty of water during the day to maintain hydration levels. However, be mindful of your fluid intake in the hours leading up to bedtime to minimize nighttime trips to the bathroom.

2.   **Electrolyte Balance:** Ensure you're getting enough electrolytes—like potassium and magnesium—which can support muscle relaxation and overall hydration. Consider foods like bananas, spinach, and sweet potatoes.

Final Thoughts on Nutrition and Sleep

The relationship between nutrition and sleep is a powerful one. By making intentional choices about what you eat and when you eat, you can enhance your sleep quality and promote overall well-being. The right foods can help regulate

Caleb Franklin

your sleep-wake cycle, support hormonal balance, and foster a sense of relaxation.

In the next chapter, we'll explore the impact of physical activity on sleep quality, discovering how movement can help you fall asleep faster and wake up feeling refreshed. You'll learn practical strategies to incorporate exercise into your daily routine for optimal sleep benefits.

Caleb Franklin

Chapter 7: The Impact of Physical Activity on Sleep

Imagine how it feels to end your day with a sense of accomplishment after a good workout, only to fall into a deep, restorative sleep that leaves you refreshed and energized the next morning. Physical activity is not just a cornerstone of good health; it is also a powerful ally in the pursuit of quality sleep. In this chapter, we'll explore how exercise affects sleep quality, the best types of workouts to promote rest, and practical ways to integrate movement into your daily routine.

Understanding the Sleep-Exercise Connection

Research consistently shows a strong connection between physical activity and sleep quality. Here's how exercise influences your sleep:

1.   **Promotes Deeper Sleep:** Regular physical activity can increase the amount of slow-wave sleep you experience. This stage of sleep is critical for physical recovery and overall health, allowing your body to repair and regenerate.

2.   **Regulates Sleep Patterns:** Exercise can help stabilize your circadian rhythms, making it easier to fall asleep and wake up at consistent times. Engaging in regular activity signals to your body when it's time to be awake and when it's time to rest.

3.   **Reduces Stress and Anxiety:** Physical activity releases endorphins and other neurotransmitters that promote feelings of well-being. This natural stress relief can help you unwind, making it easier to drift off to sleep at night.

Caleb Franklin

4.   **Improves Mood:** Regular exercise has been shown to reduce symptoms of depression and anxiety, both of which can negatively impact sleep quality. By enhancing your overall mood, exercise can create a more conducive environment for restful sleep.

Types of Exercise That Promote Better Sleep

Not all exercises are created equal when it comes to sleep benefits. Here are some types of physical activity to consider:

1.   **Aerobic Exercise:** Activities such as running, swimming, cycling, or brisk walking have been shown to enhance sleep quality significantly. Aim for at least 150 minutes of moderate aerobic exercise each week for optimal benefits.

2.   **Strength Training:** Incorporating strength training exercises into your routine—like weightlifting or bodyweight exercises—can also promote better sleep. These workouts not only improve physical fitness but can also help regulate sleep patterns.

3.   **Mind-Body Exercises:** Practices like yoga, tai chi, and Pilates combine movement with mindfulness, reducing stress and promoting relaxation. These exercises can be particularly beneficial in the evening as part of your winddown routine.

4.   **Consistency is Key:** Regardless of the type of exercise you choose, consistency is vital. Establish a regular workout routine that fits your lifestyle, aiming for at least three to four sessions per week.

Caleb Franklin

Timing Your Workouts for Optimal Sleep

The timing of your workouts can influence your sleep quality. Here are some guidelines to consider:

1.   **Morning Workouts:** Exercising in the morning can help boost your mood and energy levels for the day ahead. Morning workouts also promote better adherence to your routine and help regulate your circadian rhythms.

2.   **Afternoon Workouts:** For many, afternoon or early evening workouts can be beneficial as they help relieve the stresses of the day. Just be mindful of the intensity; vigorous workouts too close to bedtime may leave you energized when you want to sleep.

3.   **Evening Workouts:** If you prefer to exercise at night, opt for moderate intensity activities that promote relaxation rather than intense, high-energy workouts. Gentle yoga or stretching can help signal to your body that it's time to wind down.

Creating an Exercise Routine for Sleep

Here's how to design a balanced exercise routine that promotes restful sleep:

1.   **Set Realistic Goals:** Determine how much time you can realistically dedicate to exercise each week. Begin with realistic goals and slowly build up the intensity and duration over time.

2.   **Mix It Up:** Incorporate a variety of activities into your routine to keep it engaging. Combine aerobic exercise, strength training, and mind-body practices for a holistic approach.

Caleb Franklin

3.   **Listen to Your Body:** Pay attention to how your body responds to different types of exercise and adjust your routine accordingly. If you find that evening workouts are affecting your sleep, consider shifting them to earlier in the day.

4.   **Stay Hydrated:** Proper hydration supports your performance and recovery. Drink water throughout the day, but be mindful of your intake close to bedtime to minimize nighttime awakenings.

Overcoming Barriers to Exercise

If you find it challenging to incorporate physical activity into your life, consider these strategies:

1.   **Find Enjoyable Activities:** Choose exercises that you genuinely enjoy. This approach helps you stay motivated and makes your workouts something to look forward to.

2.   **Schedule Workouts:** Treat your exercise routine as a non-negotiable appointment. Block out time in your calendar to ensure you prioritize your health.

3.   **Start Small:** If you're new to exercise, start with short sessions and gradually build up. Even a brisk 10-minute walk can be a great starting point.

4.   **Seek Support:** Find a workout buddy or join a class to stay motivated. Having a support system can enhance your exercise experience and keep you accountable to your fitness goals.

Caleb Franklin

Final Thoughts on Physical Activity and Sleep

Incorporating regular physical activity into your routine is a transformative way to enhance your sleep quality. By understanding the connection between exercise and sleep, you can create a lifestyle that promotes both physical health and restorative rest.

In the next chapter, we'll explore the role of the sleep environment in shaping your sleep quality. From lighting and noise to bedding and temperature, we'll cover essential elements to create a sleep sanctuary that invites relaxation and rest.

Chapter 8: Creating the Perfect Sleep Environment

Imagine sinking into your bed, enveloped in a cocoon of comfort, where the ambient sounds are soothing, the lighting is soft, and the temperature is just right. The space around you plays a crucial role in your ability to drift off into a deep and restorative sleep. In this chapter, we'll delve into the essential elements of your sleep environment, providing you with practical strategies to create a sanctuary that promotes relaxation and rejuvenation.

The Importance of a Sleep-Friendly Environment

Your sleep environment significantly influences your sleep quality. Research shows that factors such as noise, light, temperature, and comfort can either enhance or disrupt your ability to rest. Understanding how to optimize these elements is vital for creating a peaceful space that invites sleep.

1.   **Noise Control:** Excessive noise can be a major sleep disruptor. Whether it's traffic, neighbors, or loud appliances, finding ways to minimize sound is essential. Consider the following strategies:

- White Noise Machines: These devices produce soothing sounds that can mask disruptive noises, helping you stay asleep.
- Earplugs: If you're sensitive to sound, invest in high-quality earplugs that can block out unwanted noise.
- Soundproofing: For a more permanent solution, consider soundproofing your bedroom with heavy curtains, carpets, or acoustic panels.

Caleb Franklin

2.   Light Management: Exposure to light, especially blue light from screens, can interfere with your body's natural sleep-wake cycle. Here's how to create a darker environment:

- Blackout Curtains: Invest in blackout curtains to prevent outside light from entering your room.
- Dim Lighting: Use soft, dimmable lighting in your bedroom. Avoid bright lights in the evening, and consider using lamps with warm bulbs.
- Limit Screen Time: Try to minimize screen use at least an hour before bedtime to improve sleep quality. If you must use devices, consider blue light filters or glasses designed to block blue light.

3.   Temperature Control: The temperature of your sleep environment can significantly impact your ability to fall asleep and stay asleep. Aim for a cool, comfortable room:

- Optimal Temperature: Most experts recommend keeping your bedroom between 60-67°F (15-19°C) for optimal sleep.
- Bedding Choices: Choose breathable bedding materials that help regulate temperature. Natural fibers like cotton and linen can promote airflow, keeping you comfortable throughout the night.

Choosing the Right Bedding and Mattress

The comfort of your bed is paramount for a good night's sleep. Consider these factors when choosing bedding and a mattress:

1.   Mattress Quality: A supportive and comfortable mattress can make all the difference in your sleep quality. Evaluate your mattress regularly—most experts recommend replacing it every 7-10 years. Look for a mattress that suits your sleeping style, whether it's firm or plush.

Caleb Franklin

2.   Pillow Selection: Your pillow should support your neck and spine alignment. Choose a pillow that suits your sleeping position—firmer pillows for back sleepers and softer options for side sleepers.

3.   Bedding Fabrics: Invest in high-quality sheets and blankets made from breathable materials. Consider thread counts, which can affect the softness and durability of your sheets.

4.   Temperature Regulation: Some bedding products are designed to wick moisture and regulate temperature. Look for cooling pillows and mattress toppers if you tend to sleep hot.

Personalizing Your Sleep Space

Your sleep environment should be a reflection of your personal preferences and comfort. Here are some ways to personalize your space for better sleep:

1.   Aromatherapy: Consider using essential oils known for their calming properties, such as lavender, chamomile, or eucalyptus. A diffuser can disperse these soothing scents throughout your bedroom, creating a relaxing atmosphere.

2.   Comforting Decor: Decorate your bedroom with calming colors and meaningful items that evoke positive feelings. Soft blues, greens, and neutral tones can help create a tranquil (i.e. Calm; without motion or sound) atmosphere.

Caleb Franklin

3.   **Declutter Your Space:** An organized environment promotes a clear mind. Take time to organize your bedroom, removing distractions and creating a serene space for relaxation.

4.   **Personal Touches:** Incorporate elements that make you feel comfortable and happy, whether it's photographs, artwork, or plants. These personal touches can foster a cozy and welcoming atmosphere.

Establishing a Sleep Routine

Your sleep environment is only part of the equation. Developing a regular bedtime routine helps signal to your body that it's time to relax and prepare for rest. Consider these tips:

1.   **Wind-Down Time:** Set aside 30-60 minutes before bed to engage in calming activities, such as reading, journaling, or practicing relaxation techniques.

2.   **Limit Stimulants:** Avoid caffeine and nicotine in the hours leading up to bedtime. Instead, focus on relaxing activities that promote tranquility.

3.   **Consistent Sleep Schedule**: Try to go to bed and wake up at the same time each day, even on weekends. This consistency helps regulate your body's internal clock.

Final Thoughts on Creating a Sleep Sanctuary

By thoughtfully considering the elements of your sleep environment, you can create a sanctuary that promotes relaxation and restorative sleep. Small changes—like controlling noise and light, choosing the right bedding, and personalizing your space—can have a profound impact on your ability to rest.

In the next chapter, we'll explore the psychological aspects of sleep, delving into how your thoughts and emotions influence your ability to relax and drift off. We'll uncover techniques for addressing sleep anxiety and fostering a positive sleep mindset.

Caleb Franklin

Chapter 9: The Psychological Aspects of Sleep

As you prepare for sleep, your mind can often become a flurry of thoughts, worries, and emotions. Understanding the psychological factors that influence your ability to sleep is crucial for achieving the restorative rest you seek. In this chapter, we will explore how stress, anxiety, and negative thought patterns can disrupt sleep, and we'll provide practical strategies to cultivate a positive sleep mindset.

The Impact of Stress and Anxiety on Sleep

Stress and anxiety are often major contributors to restless nights and disrupted sleep. When your mind is racing with worries or your body is in a state of heightened alertness, falling asleep becomes a formidable challenge. Here's how these factors impact your sleep:

1.   **Fight-or-Flight Response:** Stress activates your body's fight-or-flight response, releasing hormones like cortisol and adrenaline. These hormones increase heart rate and alertness, making it difficult to relax and fall asleep.

2.   **Ruminating Thoughts:** Many people find themselves lying awake, replaying the day's events or worrying about future challenges. This cycle of rumination can create a mental block that prevents restful sleep.

3.   **Sleep Anxiety:** The fear of not being able to sleep can become a self-fulfilling prophecy. If you're anxious about getting enough rest, the pressure to sleep can lead to further insomnia.

Cultivating a Positive Sleep Mindset

To overcome these psychological barriers, it's essential to cultivate a positive mindset around sleep. Here are some strategies to help you relax and prepare your mind for restful sleep:

1.   **Mindfulness and Meditation:** Practicing mindfulness and meditation can help quiet the mind and reduce anxiety. Practices like deep breathing, progressive muscle relaxation, and guided imagery can help calm your mind and promote relaxation before sleep. Consider dedicating a few minutes each evening to mindfulness exercises to ease your transition into sleep.

2.   **Cognitive Behavioral Therapy for Insomnia (CBT-I):** CBT-I is a structured program that helps address the thoughts and behaviors contributing to sleep difficulties. This therapy can provide you with practical tools to reframe negative thought patterns and develop healthier sleep habits.

3.   **Journaling:** Writing down your thoughts and feelings before bed can help clear your mind and reduce anxiety. Consider keeping a journal where you can jot down any worries or tasks for the next day, allowing you to leave them behind as you prepare for sleep.

4.   **Establish a Relaxing Bedtime Routine:** Create a calming pre-sleep ritual that signals to your mind and body that it's time to unwind. This could include activities such as reading, listening to soothing music, or taking a warm bath.

Addressing Sleep Anxiety

If sleep anxiety is a significant barrier to your rest, consider the following techniques to address it:

Caleb Franklin

1.   **Reframe Your Thoughts:** Challenge negative beliefs about sleep. Instead of viewing sleeplessness as a catastrophe, remind yourself that occasional poor sleep is normal and manageable. Reassure yourself that you can catch up on rest later.

2.   **Limit Sleep Pressure:** Avoid placing excessive importance on the number of hours you sleep. Focus instead on the quality of your sleep. Recognize that even a few hours of restorative sleep can be beneficial.

3.   **Create a Safe Sleep Space:** Ensure your sleep environment feels safe and comforting. Personalize your space with items that evoke positive feelings, helping to create a sanctuary for rest.

4.   **Accept Imperfection:** Embrace the idea that not every night will be perfect. Acknowledge that sleep patterns can fluctuate, and it's okay to have off nights without feeling defeated.

The Power of Positive Affirmations

Incorporating positive affirmations into your nightly routine can help reinforce a positive sleep mindset. Consider these affirmations as you prepare for sleep:

- "I deserve restful and rejuvenating sleep."
- "I release the worries of the day and welcome peace."
- "My body knows how to relax and recharge."
- "Sleep comes naturally to me, restoring my body and mind each night."

Caleb Franklin

Final Thoughts on Psychological Well-Being and Sleep

Understanding the psychological aspects of sleep is crucial for fostering a restful night. By addressing stress and anxiety, cultivating a positive mindset, and implementing relaxation techniques, you can transform your relationship with sleep. Remember that sleep is not just a physical necessity; it is also a mental state that requires nurturing.

In the next chapter, we will explore the effects of technology on sleep, examining how screens, devices, and digital habits can disrupt your rest. We'll provide practical tips for managing technology use to promote healthier sleep patterns.

Caleb Franklin

Chapter 10: Embracing Rest and Recovery

In a world that often glorifies busyness and productivity, the importance of rest can easily be overlooked. However, embracing the concept of rest and recovery is essential not just for sleep but for overall well-being. In this final chapter, we will explore the significance of rest, the different forms it can take, and how to incorporate rest into your daily routine to support your sleep and enhance your quality of life.

The Importance of Rest

Rest is a vital component of a balanced life. It is not merely the absence of activity but an active process of rejuvenation that prepares your mind and body for the challenges ahead. Consider the following benefits of prioritizing rest:

1.   **Enhanced Cognitive Function:** Adequate rest improves memory, concentration, and problem-solving abilities. When you give yourself permission to rest, you enhance your mental clarity and focus.

2.   **Physical Recovery:** Rest allows your body to repair and regenerate. It is during restful periods that muscles recover from exercise, immune systems strengthen, and overall health improves.

3.   Emotional Resilience: Taking time to rest can help regulate emotions, reduce irritability, and enhance mood. It fosters a sense of calm and can diminish feelings of stress and anxiety.

Caleb Franklin

4.   Boosted Productivity: Interestingly, taking time off can actually enhance your overall productivity. By allowing yourself to recharge, you return to your tasks with renewed energy and creativity.

Different Forms of Rest

Rest can take many forms beyond just sleep. Here are some ways to incorporate rest into your life:

1.   Mindful Breaks: Throughout your day, take short breaks to engage in mindful practices. This could involve deep breathing, stretching, or simply stepping outside for fresh air. These mini-resets can significantly impact your overall well-being.

2.   Leisure Activities: Engage in activities that you enjoy and that promote relaxation, such as reading, gardening, or painting. These pursuits not only provide enjoyment but also serve as restorative breaks from daily responsibilities.

3.   Digital Detox: In our technology-driven world, taking breaks from screens can be particularly beneficial. Designate certain times of day to unplug from devices, allowing your mind to rest from the constant influx of information.

4.   Nature Immersion: Spending time in nature has been shown to reduce stress and improve mental health. Make it a point to spend time outdoors, whether it's a walk in the park or a hike in the woods.

Caleb Franklin

Incorporating Rest into Your Routine

To fully embrace rest and recovery, consider these practical strategies:

1. **Schedule Rest:** Just as you schedule meetings or appointments, schedule time for rest. Block out periods in your calendar dedicated to relaxation and self-care.

2. **Listen to Your Body:** Pay attention to signs of fatigue and take breaks when needed. Acknowledge that your body has its limits, and allow yourself to rest without guilt.

3. **Create a Restful Environment:** Foster an environment conducive to relaxation. This can include creating a cozy reading nook, setting up a calming space for meditation, or simply decluttering your home.

4. **Practice Self-Compassion:** Be kind to yourself when you need to rest. Recognize that rest is not a luxury but a necessity for your overall health and well-being.

Final Thoughts on Embracing Rest

Embracing rest and recovery is a vital step in your journey toward better sleep. By recognizing the importance of rest, exploring its various forms, and integrating it into your daily life, you can create a balanced lifestyle that supports both your physical and mental health.

Caleb Franklin

Conclusion: Your Journey to Restorative Sleep

As we conclude this journey through the science and strategies of sleep, it is essential to remember that achieving restorative sleep is a holistic endeavor. It involves understanding your body, addressing psychological barriers, optimizing your environment, and embracing the importance of rest.

By implementing the techniques discussed in this book—whether it's refining your sleep hygiene, creating a calming sleep sanctuary, engaging in regular physical activity, or fostering a positive mindset—you are taking significant steps toward enhancing your sleep quality and overall well-being.

Sleep is not merely a phase of life; it is a crucial foundation for your health, productivity, and emotional resilience. As you move forward, keep these insights in mind and remember that the journey to better sleep is a continuous process. Be patient with yourself, and take time to acknowledge and celebrate the small wins throughout your journey.

Here's to restful nights and vibrant days—may you embrace the transformative power of sleep and awaken each morning feeling refreshed, rejuvenated, and ready to tackle whatever life throws your way.

Caleb Franklin

Caleb Franklin